Coconut Oil for Health and Beauty

The Ultimate Guide to using Coconut Oil for Healthy Hair, Glowing Skin, Incredible Weight Loss and More!

Sarah Lillard

Table of Contents

Introduction

Once upon a time, not so very long ago, there were medical professionals who gave out a decree on the status of coconut oil. With its high saturated fat content, the royalty of medicine declared, coconut oil couldn't possibly be good for the human body. It was banished to the land in which no person would dare enter without risking their health.

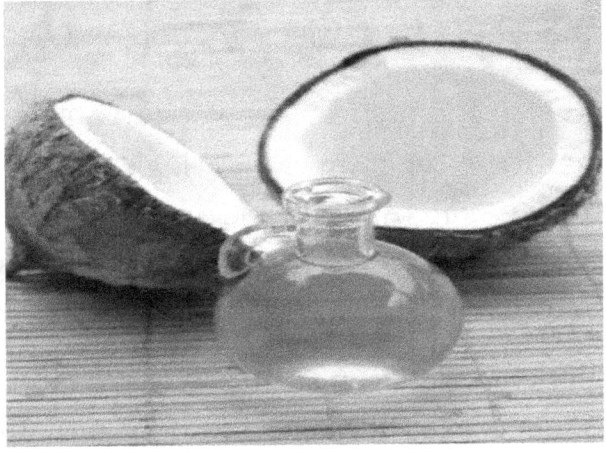

The royalty of medical care walked away and it was presumed everyone lived happily ever after.

Not so fast there! As with everything in the real world, nothing is a safe bet except, ironically, change.

Soon there was another generation of medical royalty ascending the throne, continuing to research areas that others – yourself in fact – considered closed to discussion years ago.

Though the above presentation is unconventional way introducing you to the benefit of coconut oil, you certainly understand the idea behind it. Someone, somewhere, took another look at this often-used ingredient from a different angle. They looked once more at the health potential of this oil despite its high saturated fat content. Something they read, perhaps, triggered a question about this oil.

If science and especially health matters were static endeavors that never changed, what would be the fun in studying them? It wouldn't be an adventure. And that brave person would never have dared entered that dense, dark forest of banished studies. Now is the time to revisit a topic that was once thought to be settled for good and overturn a decreed verdict.

Before you read this book overcome with an attitude of hardcore cynicism wondering what's wrong with the medical community to even think of overlooking the healthy benefits of something as simple as coconut oil, be thankful that we live in a world that has a scientific community that's willing – and indeed eager – to continue to push forward with research in a seeking ever healthier methods of eating and living.

Part of the reason for what seems to be a merry-go-round of opinions on the topic, along with other health-related subjects, is the recognition that health is much more complicated than any of us can ever imagine. If there were a recipe you could follow – a set of instructions -- that would 100 percent guarantee we could live to be 90 or 100 or any preset age you'd like placed on the "guarantee protection sheet," then you would know where you stood! You would know exactly what combination of foods absolutely ensured a long and healthy life free from degenerative diseases.

A Second Look at Coconut Oil

Alas! There isn't. That means the search for the healthiest ways to live continue to be researched. A segment of the medical community seeks out even more evidence concerning topics many laypersons thought were written in stone. Coconut oil is simply one more example of this.

If by chance, you're one of the many individuals who hasn't yet heard about coconut oil – either when it was deemed bad or now when it's gaining favor once more – you'll be pleased to learn about a new, versatile oil that's used in everything from cooking to cosmetics.

If, on the other hand, you're taking a second look at this oil, you'll be amazed at its newfound potential to help you create the healthiest – and most beautiful – you possible. At least I certainly hope so. Why? Because this book is nothing less than a labor of love for me.

I wrote this book because I've benefitted firsthand from the health benefits of coconut oil. I've gone from cynic ("Yeah, right!" I would say sarcastically when someone would praise this oil) – to open minded to . . . yes, you guessed it . . a proponent of coconut oil as a healthy addition to your diet and lifestyle.

I'll spare you all the details, but I will explain that several years ago I was woefully overweight, fighting constant fatigue and was indifferent to everything in my life. I knew something was wrong. I visited my personal health care provider. She gave me a battery of tests. She took so much blood out of me for testing I was beginning to think she was a vampire and asked me so many questions I thought she was grilling me about the murder of the century.

Needless to say my doctor worked hard for her money, but could find absolutely nothing wrong with me. My blood tests came back and apparently I was eating well. While I was grateful for all of her hard work, I was supremely disappointed that she couldn't find out what was wrong with me.

In fact, at this point, I really was beyond discovering *what* was wrong with me. I just wanted to "fix" it. I wanted to feel more energetic. I wanted my old life back – and quickly.

Finally I met a friend for coffee one day shortly after that series of tests. She knew something was wrong even before I told her.

I explained I didn't know and apparently neither did the doctor. "But is it so bad you can tell just by looking at me?" I asked.

"Your hair isn't as shiny or healthy-looking as it usually is," she began. "Not only that, your skin used to have a type of glow to it – and it just doesn't any more. Are you under stress?"

"No more than usual," I said.

"Sometimes, after we've been deluged with stress and insist on running around doing everything without resting, we don't realize the toll it takes on our bodies. Trust me, I've done that before," she said.

I nodded my head. That certainly could have been me, I thought. "You look great, though," I said. "What's your secret?"

She never even hesitated to share it with me. "Coconut oil."

Of course, I wasn't quite ready to accept it at that point. I looked at her incredulously. "Really?"

"I wouldn't kid about anything like that," she said. "Then she proceeded to tell me about all the great new things people are saying about coconut oil."

"I thought it was high in saturated fats," I said. That's all I could think to say. It was, actually all I knew of coconut oil.

"But more importantly," my friend continued as she took a sip of her coffee, "I found a doctor who knew a lot of the latest studies on coconut oil. He urged me to give it a try. Why don't I send you his phone number and some of the web sites he urged me to check out?"

I thanked her, but didn't wait for her recommendations. I swear I nearly ran home and began checking out everything I could about coconut oil. After all, what did I have to lose?

I eventually saw her doctor, but by the time I had an appointment, I was knee-deep in articles about coconut oil and learning lots of ways of using itnot only in my daily diet, but also in my daily beauty routine as well.

By the time I finally met with her doctor I was actually beginning to feel better. I told him I had begun using coconut oil – for cooking, for cleansing my skin, even in my shampoo. He agreed that it was undoubtedly contributing to the betterment of my health.

Today . . . .

I am healthier, more energetic and happier than I've ever been – and in my eyes I owe it all to my versatile use of coconut oil. And now I feel as if I want to tell the entire world exactly how I did it.

I want everyone to be able to duplicate my come-back story. If you're feeling sluggish, not up to your usual self, think about the possibility that you're missing some essential nutrients that coconut oil can provide.

In the coming chapters, I'll explain exactly what coconut oil and how you can use it to your greater advantage. Not only that, but we'll talk about some of these amazing topics:

- How coconut oil can help keep degenerative diseases like heart disease and diabetes at bay
- Learn to use coconut oil to your advantage if you've tried losing weight and failed even though you're following all the rules
- Discover 40 ways to incorporate coconut oil in your diet and your daily beauty routine
- Find out what types of coconut oil are available and their most advantageous uses
- Discover why coconut oil pulling is gaining in popularity and how it can increase your health exponentially

- And much, much more!

How to Use This Book

It's totally up to you how you read through and eventually use this book. But I've written it so that you can learn the most important scientific facts, research studies and exciting successful uses of other dedicated coconut oil consumers. You'll probably want to read through the entire book at least once.

After that you may desire to choose your toughest health issues and apply coconut oil to working on these issues. Need to lose weight? Then after reading the entire book, don't hesitate to make a beeline to that chapter and adapt the knowledge found there to your needs.

You may be tempted to change your life in a half dozen ways all at once. Resist that urge. Work on one area at a time. If it's weight – then concentrate on using this amazing oil for losing weight. While you're doing this, you'll discover something totally astounding happening – other health areas of your life will slowly recover and eventually blossom healthy and energetically.

Are you ready to discover the near miraculous health giving secrets of coconut oil? Are you tired of feeling tired, feeling cheated out of the best years of your life and missing some of the most vital activities of your children?

Who else wants to take back their life? Regain the energy they thought they lost and in the process protect their health from increased risks of heart disease, diabetes, even Alzheimer's and more?

Then follow me to Chapter 1 and I'll tell you about just a few of the many ways coconut oil can play a critical role in your health.

Chapter 1: Coconut Oil Claims

If you're still cynical and remain unconvinced about the health benefits of coconut oil, then you'll be interested in reading the rest of this chapter. I certainly don't expect you to take my word for the effectiveness of this amazing oil. But I have culled the web and professional medical journals where documentation of these benefits exists.

I've also talked to natural health care providers, health food

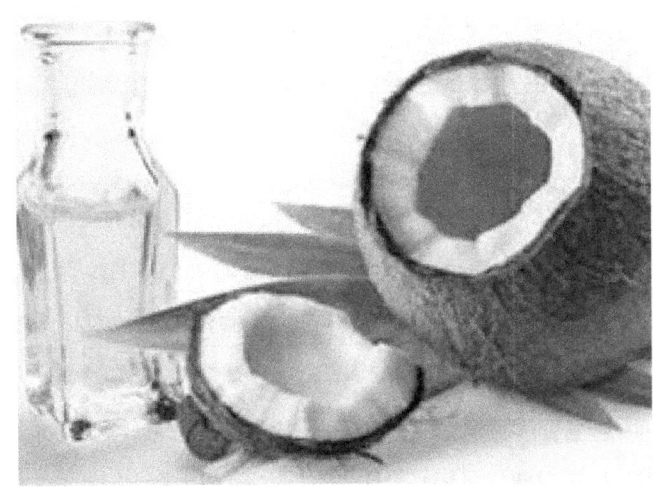 store owners and others intimate with the uses of natural health tools. Throughout this chapter you'll discover details of the studies, and professionals' ideas on coconut oil.

Immune System, Thyroid and Glucose Levels, Oh My!

Studies, in fact, now indicate that the once-overlooked coconut oil can help your immune system defend itself against bacterial invasion as well as viral attacks on your body. What does that mean to your overall health? It means you may find yourself experiencing less sickness and illness throughout the year. It means in a nutshell, you may very well be the person who stays healthy in the middle of the flu or colds are attacking and keep everyone else in bed.

But with a heightened immune system, it appears, according to the latest research, that using coconut oil just may be the key to help you ward off other infections as well, specifically **yeast, fungus and candida.**

Coconut oil may also play a role in affecting your **endocrine system.** It's been noted that those individuals who use this substance regularly discover the hormones controlling both their **thyroid glands** and their **glucose levels.** Thyroid hormone levels can affect your energy level – either for better or worse. And of course, it's widely known that glucose levels are the most effective way of diagnosing diabetes.

Coconut Oil and Cholesterol Levels

Here's the $64,000 question: how can any oil that is overwhelmingly drenched in saturated fats possibly be expected to reduce cholesterol levels? The answer lies in the type of fatty acid in this oil. Coconut oil contains a saturated fat that's referred to as a lauric acid. This variety of acid, in turn, is considered a type of MCT – a medium chain triglyceride.

The good news is that this MCT helps to increase the "good" or HDL cholesterol in your blood. Because of its presence, the coconut oil actually aids in improving the ultimate cholesterol ratio levels.

The use of coconut oil on a regular basis helps to lower cholesterol by converting it to pregnenolone. I know this probably means little to you, but it's a molecule that's a precursor to many of the hormones your body demands on a daily basis in order to keep it humming along efficiently.

Now, let's just return to the mention of your thyroid gland earlier. If you use coconut oil regularly you may discern that because of your raised energy level, your thyroid is beginning to function at normal levels once more. But wait, there's more. Because health is seldom isolated, the thyroid gland, functioning normally, in turn helps to reduce your levels of bad or LDL cholesterol levels.

Coconut Oil and Alzheimer's Disease

It's the enigma of the twenty-first century – Alzheimer's disease. It seems to attack people randomly. While usually affecting the older individual, persons as young as 50 have been known to be at risk for, and actually displayed symptoms of, the "early onset" version of this heart-breaking disorder.

While there are tips and suggestions to help prevent it, there are no guarantees that you will live the rest of your life with your full memory intact. It's a scary disorder for the entire family – the individual affected directly with it and those who have to take care of their loved one.

Now, there appears to be a bright star on the horizon regarding the prevention of this insipid disease. Yes, it really does come in the form of coconut oil. And Dr. Mary Newport is probably one of the most enthusiastic proponents of it.

Her husband, who has suffered from Alzheimer's disease since he was 51, dramatically improved after just a short time on this regime. It's just part of the story she tells in her 2011 book, ***Alzheimer's Disease: What If There Was a Cure? The Story of Ketones.***

She's not the only medical professional who's taking note of coconut oil and memory loss. Recently, the University of Oxford conducted research that reveals the improvement is only temporary. Keep in mind that coconut oil at least helps for a short time.

The Oxford study and Dr. Newport's own research align nicely. Dr. Newport theorizes that as the fats break down in your body, by products of this process, called ketones, are crucial in maintaining brain health. The underlying idea is that as you boost the number of ketones in your body, which are found in coconut oil, you can indeed help to improve your brain health.

Four Ways Coconut Oil Aids Liver Function

Okay, I realize the liver is not an exciting organ to learn about – let alone an exciting subject. But it is a vital organ, far more important in our metabolism and other areas of health than most of us realize. It's heartening then to learn that the regular use of coconut oil can help the healthy functioning of your liver in essential five ways.

1. Helps to Convert Energy

The seemingly magical work of coconut oil helps to convert what you eat into energy before it hits the liver, relieving the organ of quite a bit of work. This is where those medium chain triglycerides found in the oil – as well as other fatty acids – come into play.

Specifically, the scientific studies center on the role of medium chain triglycerides – which are found in coconut oil – fatty acids and the prevention of live disease. MCT and fatty acids are readily transformed into energy upon reaching the liver.

That being the case, this process then helps to reduce the pressure on the liver. It, in effect, has to work less.

2. Prevents the accumulation of fat

This process, by the way, also aids in the prevention of the accumulation of fat.

3. Improves Your Metabolism

Did you know that health professionals consider coconut oil antiviral, antibacterial and antifungal? Because of these characteristics, steady use of this oil helps to boost your metabolism. Again, you can thank the medium chain fatty acids in the oil. It's their presence that allows your body to deal basically a death blows to microbes.

4. Stifles free radical development

Once again this result of the use of coconut oil is due to the medium chain fatty acids we've been talking about. The latest round of scientific research reveals that thanks to its ability slowing of free radical development, daily coconut oil use may actually reduce a person's risk of alcohol-induced liver damage.

Holy Weight Loss!

I promised you we'd talk about coconut oil and weight loss. We'll continue this discussion in an upcoming chapter devoted to weight loss, but for the moment, here are some statistics and research results to keep in mind.

Remember that MCT we talked about just a few paragraphs ago. You can thank that substance for the ability of coconut oil to maintain a balanced weight. Recent research vividly illustrates that exposure MCT in this oil helps to break down this type of triglyceride and eventually aids in the accumulation of healthy fats in the liver. The bottom line? This means the liver can more efficiently burn energy to speed the process of burning energy – sometimes also known as your metabolism rate.

Let's look at one study about this from several years ago. It was conducted back in 2009, but it's still relevant today. Women who consumed approximately two (2) tablespoons of coconut oil a day for three months didn't gain weight. Not only that, but these females actually reduced the amounts of their abdominal fat, specifically, the type of fat that is not only more difficult than normal to shed, but the type whose presence leads to a greater risk of acquiring heart problems.

Coconut Oil and the Aging Process!

Yes, it's true. But this really shouldn't come as much of a surprise. We've already hinted at this amazing oil and how it can help protect you from such diseases as diabetes and heart disease. These are just two of the degenerative diseases that can easily lead a person to a faster rate of aging.

So it only is logical that more than one researcher has discovered that coconut oil contributes to the reduction of the aging process. No, it's no fountain of youth by a long shot, but if it could help keep the process in check, that's a good thing.

How does it do this? By exerting a positive antioxidant affect in your body. In effect, taking coconut oil regularly can actually help to slow – and in some cases even halt – the damage to other healthy fats and tissues in your body.

Coconut oil slows the rate of oxidation in your body, which is the major cause, according to the medical community, of cardiovascular disorders as well as aging skin. Let's just make this clear: When you use coconut oil on a regular basis you're actually helping your body to be less dependent on antioxidant consumption.

Impressive, isn't it?

Healthy Hair

Don't get me wrong. Warding off, thwarting and keeping those degenerative diseases at bay goes a long way to slowing the aging process. But there's another – no less exciting way – that will help keep that youthful look in your appearance.

That's through careful selection your health and beauty products. Coconut oil, in recent years, is being recognized as a marvelous moisturizer for both your hair and your skin. You've probably noticed it yourself. It's hard not to. Whenever you step into the health and beauty department of any store, you're well aware that nearly every shampoo and body soap try to outdo the others with the print equivalent of shouting it contains coconut oil.

When you add vitamin E to the recipe – a highly effective antioxidant in its own right -- then you're looking at a powerful anti-aging beauty product.

But just be sure that if you're using this particular shampoo regularly or series of various brands of shampoos with coconut oil, that you double check that the product is made from *organic coconut oil.* It will make all the difference in the world.

It's Never Too Early . . .

At least that's the advice of many coconut oil proponents. They heartily advise parents of newly born infants to massage their little bodies with coconut oil following a bath. And yes, there are some statistics to show that this provides your child with untold eventual health benefits.

Convinced? But Don't Know How to Use It?

As we continue in this book, you'll become the master of substituting coconut oil for many items in your diet. Until that time comes, of course, you may be itching to get started. Even baby steps, you've decided (and rightly so!) can make great strides in the state of your health.

Eager to start? Why not try this? Here's a hint: coconut oil works its magic in both baked goods and on vegetables. Like zucchini and banana bread? There's absolutely no reason why you can't put coconut oil in your homemade versions of both of these.

Many people love kale and other bitter greens when they're drizzled with coconut oil. But don't let your imagination stop there. What if I told you I use it as part of my standard onion and garlic sauté? My family loves it so much now that when I don't use this threesome together (coconut oil, onion and garlic) my family feels cheated.

If you've never tried it then you're in for a distinctly different full-bodied taste. My family guarantees you'll fall in love with it, just like they did.

But don't neglect to bring this awesome oil for breakfast as well. Think for a moment about spreading it over your morning breakfast oatmeal. Not only can you say that you're helping to maintain your health – but you're making your morning meal more pleasurable. It's going to taste even creamier than ever. Guaranteed.

What about Adverse Side Effects?

This is the part of the chapter when I write about the potential negative side effects of the very substance I'm talking about. So what about coconut oil? you ask. Does it have any side effects?

From everything the current research indicates, coconut oil is quite safe with minimum – if any side effects. Of course, that proclamation of approval is based on the presumption that you are using moderate amounts of it. Anything – even the healthiest of substances – can have adverse side effects if you use too much.

One of the problems is that no one has yet to be able to tell us how much is too much. So it's up to each individual to carefully monitor how much he takes. But according to all the most recent research, very little is really needed to boost your health. In fact, as little as one or two teaspoons a day can transform your health. Imagine that!

Chapter 2: Healthy Skin and Hair

It just makes sense. You're feeding your body coconut oil to improve your overall health. It's got to affect the health of your skin and hair as well.

But some individuals desire to help Mother Nature along by nurturing their bodies – especially their skin and hair -- topically as well. They apply the coconut oil to 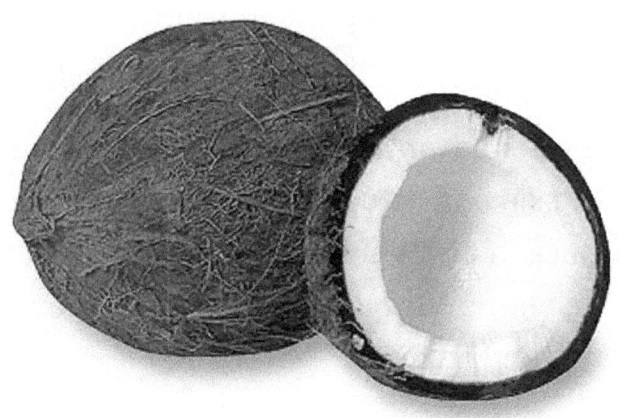 specific areas they'd like to see improve allowing all the nutrients to eventually soak in. The bottom line of this approach is that it works.

Whether you start from the inside out or the "outside in" you'll discover that coconut oil provides you with a myriad of health benefits. As such, there really are few limits of how it can work its wonders.

According to celebrity nutritionist Kimberly Snyder, who spent years traveling the world checking out natural beauty treatments, "commercial moisturizers contain lots of water, which makes you feel like your skin is being moisturized."

But she admits that's really not the case. The moment the water is wiped away or evaporates, "your skin becomes dry again."

Additionally, she asserts, many of the commercial brands of moisturizers are made with petroleum-based products, which do nothing more than suffocate your skin.

In contrast, when you use coconut oil or your own homemade blend of natural ingredients including this oil, you're actually providing your body with a deep, long-lasting moisturizer.

The clear advantage to this is that coconut oil absorbs into your skin and actually strengthens the tissues below the surface. It also helps to get rid of the excessive dead skin cells lying on the surface of the skin. The dead cells make your skin rough and flaky.

When used as a shampoo or scalp rub, you can count on coconut oil to give your hair a shine it probably hasn't had since you were a kid. It can also work as an efficient, natural moisturizer for your hair as well.

Buying Coconut Oil-Containing Products

You may already have some hair and skin products containing coconut oil. It's hard to pick any health or beauty aid off the shelf and *not* find coconut oil in it. But, now that you're becoming coconut-oil savvy, you'll want to be discriminating in the quality of the product you purchase.

The first rule of thumb in selecting health and beauty aids with this vital ingredient is to look for the words "extra virgin," Snyder advises. You can be sure that this variety "has not been hydrogenated, bleached, refined or deodorized."

Select only products labeled "organic." This ensures that the coconut oil is not genetically modified. You'll receive the best results, i.e., the healthiest possible hair, by using coconut oil that has not been refined or otherwise modified. You want to use it as close to as Mother Nature made it as possible.

One of the first questions I receive when someone buys their first bottle is "Do I have to refrigerate it?" No, you don't.

I know one of my friends keeps a bottle next to her bed, and a second bottle in the kitchen. Storing coconut oil, by the way, at a temperature lower than 76 degrees Fahrenheit solidifies it. If you store it any temperature below 76, it has a tendency to turn into a liquid.

Doctor-Approved (and Used)

Dr. Taneen Bhatia, a medical doctor specializing in integrative medicine, whole heartedly agrees with Snyder. She doesn't hesitate to point out the number of commercial beauty products which proudly list coconut oil as an ingredient. "I use it in my hair," she said, "and on my skin for deep conditioning."

Dr. Bhatia believes that coconut oil penetrates the hair deeper and easier than either mineral or sunflower oil and has the research to back up her claim. Below are several ways, Dr. Bhatia suggests that coconut oil can bring out the natural beauty – and health – in you.

1. Using it as a Hair Conditioner

She advises that when you use coconut oil as a conditioner for your hair use it before you go to bed at night. Apply a dollop of oil no larger than the size of a quarter. Rub it in, then comb your hair. After that, if your hair is long enough, pile it up on your head in a loose bun. Either wrap your head in a towel or sleep in a shower cap overnight.

In the morning you can then shampoo your hair as usual.

2. Makeup Remover

Coconut oil is a gentle, yet effective, means of removing eye makeup. Wait until you try it out on waterproof mascara – it even works wonders here!

Using a cotton ball, simply sweep it over your eyes, paying close attention to that area under your eyes as well. Be gentle in this process.

What you're going to discover is that this oil works wonders at breaking down the waxy and inky eye makeup. But perhaps the biggest surprise is that it does all this without making your skin feel dried out. Even the most delicate of areas will be hydrated. Once you've removed your makeup with the oil, then you can wash your face as usual.

3. Body Moisturizer

Coconut oil is super-effective at two things, according to a recent study. First, it's great at hydrating the skin. Second, it helps to reduce water loss in super dry skin. When something is this good at both of these aspects, you can't help but think body moisturizer. And so you should.

When you're applying this oil to your face, use it like any commercial brand of moisturizer. At first, the coconut oil will seem to have a greasier feel than probably anything else you've ever used. Give it time, though. It'll quickly absorb deep, down into your skin. Believe it or not, all you need is a spoonful of the coconut oil to moisturize your entire body.

4. As a Face Cleanser

Read that again, so you know exactly what I mean. I didn't say a moisturizer, even though we've already proved that. It's also a marvelous method of actually washing your face.

After all, we've already established that coconut oil is antifungal and antibacterial. It only makes sense it would make a safe and effective face cleanser. But it actually goes one step further than that as well.

It's great at clearing up *atopic dermatitis,* more commonly called eczema. For this reason, many women use it without fail as their only night time face moisturizer.

If you're interested in giving this a try, here's a quick and easy way to do it:

1. Using a circular motion, massage the coconut oil on your face and neck. Enjoy the massage aspect as you go.

2. Wash off the residue using your favorite cleanser.

These are only a few ways coconut oil can help keep your hair and skin youthful and healthy. There are twenty more tips, techniques and tricks on this topic, later in this book.

Now it's time to talk coconut oil and disease. Since coconut oil is a natural antibiotic and antifungal, it's not surprising that it's so effective on your health. You're about to see just how effective it really is.

Chapter 3: Say Goodbye to Degenerative Diseases

It's refreshing. But more than that, it's liberating. More modern medical doctors than ever before are allowing their patients to try natural measures to help alleviate all types of diseases before they prescribe harsh prescription medication.

That's because more patients than ever before are finally realizing that using natural health doesn't necessarily confine them to the fringes of conventional treatment.

In fact, there's even a term these days for a treatment approach that takes advantage the best of both worlds. It's

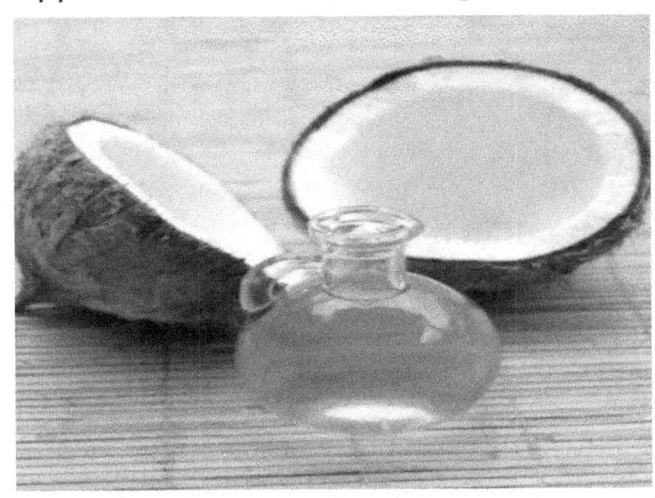

called **integrative medicine.** At one time patients who claim they've cured their depression through a structured walking program have been met with skepticism by their medical doctors.

So it's not surprising that medical doctors are now more open-minded about using different foods to help not only prevent a wide variety of diseases, but even alleviate and slow some of the symptoms.

Among these foods is the fascinating story of coconut oil. If you were just giving it nutritional label a quick glance, you'd probably shy away from it. The main reason is that you'll instantly see that it's quite high in saturated fat. This is the "bad" type of fat, usually associated with animal fats.

In fact, coconut oil contains more saturated fat than butter and is considered a solid fat. So far, this description is far from the definition of a health food. But stay with me on this one.

Before we go much farther, let's do a quick look at the nutritional numbers of one tablespoon of coconut oil:

- 117 calories

- 13.6 total fat

    o 11.8 g saturated

    o 0.8 g monounsaturated

    o 0.2 g polyunsaturated

And that's basically the entire content of coconut oil. It contains no discernible nutrients, except for trace amounts of iron and vitamins E and K and no proteins or carbohydrates.

It's similar to all the other plant-based oils you use in that it contains no cholesterol.

The real good news about coconut oil, specifically the virgin oil, is that it possesses some antioxidant properties. Researchers so far have attributed these to phenolic compounds that are commonly found in plants.

It may very well be that it's these antioxidant properties that account for its positive effects on a host of degenerative diseases.

A degenerative disease, by the way, is a disease, disorder or condition of the body caused by the wear and tear of the body as it ages. For the most, part degenerative diseases aren't infectious. Degenerative health problems are usually considered to be the collateral damage of "the normal aging process."

Examples of degenerative diseases include

- Cancer

- Chronic Obstructive Pulmonary Disease (COPD)

- Alzheimer's disease

- Atherosclerosis

- Diabetes

- Heart Disease

- Inflammatory Bowel Disease (IBD)

- Macular degeneration

- Multiple sclerosis

- Muscular dystrophy

- Osteoporosis

- Parkinson's Disease

- Prostatitis

- Rheumatoid Arthritis

Having said that, I must add that you really don't have to shrug your shoulders and accept your declining health. Not by a long shot. Medical science is making amazing strides into the specific causes of many of these health conditions. Once they know the cause, it's infinitely easier to find out the most effective methods of treating them.

For many of these diseases, regular exercise will not only delay or prevent the onset of them, but in many cases actually reverse the condition itself. When your mother would tell you when you were a child that "you are what you eat," you probably didn't take her seriously. You may not exactly be what you eat, but your health is certainly a clear reflection of your diet.

More individuals than ever before are using coconut oil in place of other less healthy varieties. Another advantage of using coconut oil is its high "smoke point." This is the upper limits of the temperature where gets too hot and burns itself along with other foods.

How to use Coconut Oil on Degenerative Diseases

One of the most effective ways of getting all the benefits of this oil is simply by cooking with it. That's right! All you really need to do is switch from your regular oil to this exotic-sounding oil. You may want to do so even if you currently believe that you're using best possible oil – olive oil.

You may find it harder than you thought to give up your currently healthy oil and enter the realm of what for you is the unknown. But once you make the switch you'll discover it'll be a part of your daily routine.

Why? Consider, first, it's very light, sweet, yet somewhat nutty coconut flavor as well as the aroma as it wafts throughout your home.

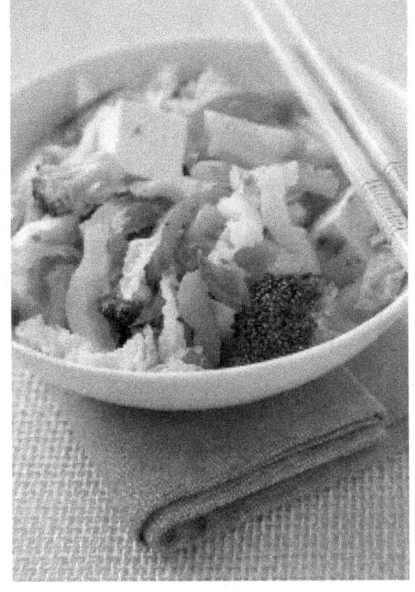

It's actually the perfect oil with which to sauté. You can turn the heat up to the medium-high setting without the worry of burning your sauté dish. You can subject this oil up to approximately 350 degrees without worrying about burning your food. This, by the way, makes it an excellent choice when you prepare curries or other foods that have just a hint of that slight tropical flavor.

If you've used the virgin oil to cook with and dislike its taste, then you can always turn to the refined coconut oil. This type is oil, is as we mentioned earlier, tasteless. That's not necessarily a bad thing when you're frying some food whose aroma and flavor can stand on its own.

Unrefined virgin oil can withstand a heating point a bit higher than the virgin. Veggies are great heated this way whether you're sautéing them on medium heat or creating a delicious Chinese stir fry dish. Unrefined coconut oil can withstand temperatures of nearly 425 degrees.

You can also substitute coconut oil for recipes calling for other kinds of oils. In this way you can receive all of its healthy benefits. It's especially an excellent option when you're seeking cooking oil that's basically flavorless.

It's an especially suitable substitute for those vegans or strict vegetarians. Since it's plant based, you'll be able to use it in place of butter which is derived from animals. And if you've ever tried to sauté or fry with butter you know firsthand then that it doesn't take a high heat for the butter to start smoking.

Believe it or not, all the coconut oil you really need to consume to make a difference in your long-term health is one to two tablespoons daily. You can easily do that through some obvious exchanges in your choice of cooking oils.

But there are plenty of other ways this can be accomplished as well. Later in this book I devote an entire chapter offering you ideas of how to incorporate this amazing oil in your diet.

But before we go there, let's talk about coconut oil and weight loss. That's the topic of the next chapter.

Chapter 4: Coconut Oil and Weight Loss

Meet your new best friend when it comes to weight loss: coconut oil. That may be a bit of an overstatement, but not by much.

There are many reasons how weight loss is heightened simply by adding coconut oil to your diet. Many of these include the addition of nutrients that help your body as well as feed many of your starving organs and tissues.

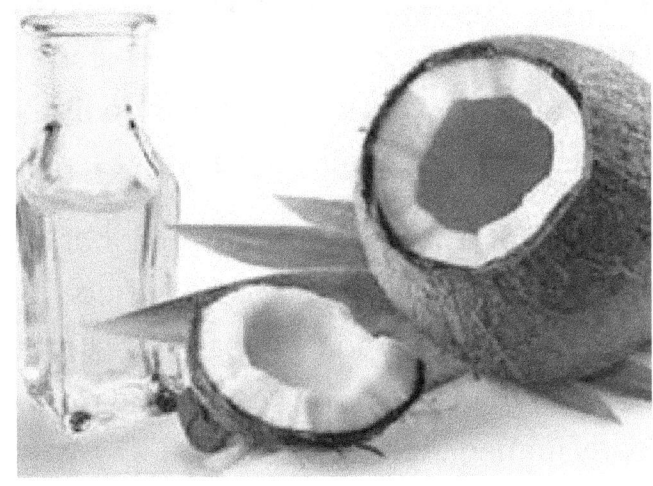

But here are just a few of the ways coconut oil can aid in your weight loss easily and near effortlessly.

1. Increased energy levels

Thanks to the medium-chain triglyceride lauric acid content of the oil, it actually affects your metabolism in a far different fashion than other oils. You'll discover the truth of this sentence once you compare your energy level after you eat something that's either been prepared with coconut oil in or has been sautéed with it than when you eat meat or dairy products.

Why? We've already talked about this briefly, but I want to make sure you know why it's energizing following a meal instead of putting you to sleep.

Your body doesn't store foods that contain medium-chain triglyceride as fat. Instead, your body responds to them by rushing them immediately to the liver. It's in this organ where the MCT content is then swiftly transformed into energy. Think of it this way: any food you eat with coconut oil in it will move its fat content directly to the head of the line to enter the liver where your body will metabolize it. Your body response to this action will be increased energy.

All other fat, those without the coconut oil, are pushed aside and are potentially headed for your body's favorite fat storage area. Think of any food you eat that contains coconut oil has a free card to move to the head of the class to be metabolized nearly immediately.

The easiest way to supercharge your metabolism: simply add two or three tablespoons of the oil to your food. You can add it to your oatmeal in the morning or your cottage cheese. If you use unrefined you can even put it in your morning smoothie without noticing any taste discrepancy.

2. Curbs your Cravings

Ah! Don't you wish there was one substance that could actually do that. What if I told you coconut oil can do just that and reduce your overall hunger as well?

Sounds too good to be true? Well, according to the latest research it really is true. Once again this is magnificent news for any individual who has every dieted or even tried to fight a craving for a specific type of food.

At the risk of sounding like a broken record, it's due once more to the medium-chain triglyceride of the oil. You'll recall that the MCT content pushes itself to the head of the line to enter the liver. And yes, because of that it gives you more energy.

But this same action . . .

Also allows your body to form something called ketones. It's these marvelous ketones that are responsible for the reduction in both hunger and food cravings. It's pretty obvious learning this, to understand why your cravings are reduced and you're finally able to lose weight a bit faster.

It takes as little as two to three tablespoons of coconut oil for this to occur. It really doesn't matter how your body receives it. In a smoothie. Through cooking your favorite foods. You decide!

3. Burn Fat Faster

Not only will you burn fat faster with coconut oil, you may also be able to digest fewer calories which equates to faster weight loss.

I tell this to many individuals who immediately worry about eating so many fewer calories without harming your health. Coconut oil is near magical in its ability to help the body digest its food faster and absorb nutrients more efficiently – all without any adverse side effects. You won't feel weak and you're not going to be tired all the time. Guaranteed!

But, there's more. Some scientific studies have discovered that coconut oil is actually a wonderful way to naturally boost your mood and actually help alleviate some of that daily stress that weighs you down.

Think, for a moment, about the long-term consequences of this fast-burning fat. Many individuals say that once they take coconut oil, they're more motivated to exercise. No, that desire won't pop up after one or even two uses of coconut oil, but it will occur. And that, in turn, will help your body burn the fat you've already stored. It's especially good at helping you drop that dangerous fat around your stomach.

All because you've been using two to three tablespoons of coconut oil daily.

4. Balance Your Hormones

As you read about all the amazing effects coconut oil has on your body, you may be realizing just what a marvellously well-oiled (no pun intended) machine your body really is. There's not an organ or a cell for that matter that works in isolation. Holistic health is indeed very real.

For your body, then, to breakdown and use the hormones of your body most efficiently it needs the fatty acids and its derivations that coconut oil possesses.

You may be tempted to dismiss the last statement. Don't. Your endocrine system, for one thing, is too important to allow mere chance to ensure it works properly.

Just take a quick glance at all the tasks it aids in the working of:

- Proper moods
- Thyroid function
- Good digestion
- Healthy sex drive
- Overall metabolism

And this list doesn't even begin to delve into how each of these areas affects even the finer points of your body's functioning.

Again, it's the medium-chain triglycerides in this oil that make this possible. The MCT content aids the body in converting the cholesterol found in your blood stream into a bio-chemical substance called pregnenoline. This substance is one of the major precursors for your body's hormones. The bottom line is that coconut oil boosts the production of your hormones, which help regulate nearly every activity of your body.

The bottom line is very good, indeed, for your weight loss goals. Using coconut oil every day makes it easier for you to lose weight in those areas where all the experts tell you it's the most dangerous: buttocks, thighs, and of course the waist.

5. Coconut Oil Efficiently Absorbs Nutrients

This healthy advantage of coconut oil goes hand-in-hand with its ability to assuage your digestive ills. Most importantly, coconut oil plays a major role in helping your system absorb fat-soluble vitamins – A, D, E, and K.

These are the nutrients tasked with responsibilities to those bodily activities we seldom think of – probably didn't even know they occurred. The fat-soluble vitamins help in promoting cellular regeneration, maintenance of healthy skin, strengthening your bones, improving your mental health and regulating brain function in general.

In addition to that, vitamin D also promotes the absorption of such health-giving minerals as calcium, zinc, iron and magnesium.

When your body possesses all the nutrients it requires, the chances are very much improved that you'll not only manage the stressors of your day better, but it'll help ward off those destructive cravings for food.

6. Coconut Oil and Your Blood Sugar

Here's one of the greatest advantages of coconut oil. Your body absorbs it without the need of digestive enzymes. This means that your pancreas needs to work less during the digestive process and instead concentrate on the more efficient production of insulin.

But, that's not all. It also helps your body's cells bind with insulin during the digestive process itself.

This can ensure that your body has the correct amount of insulin, and your cells receive the glucose, or blood sugar, they need to get your through your daily activities.

That's all well and good, you say, but how does that affect whether I lose weight or not?

When you take one or two tablespoons of coconut oil every day, then you're giving your body the tools it needs to maintain a stable glucose level. More glucose means more energy. When you have more energy, you'll want move around and . . . dare I say? . . . even exercise some.

But even more than that the potential coconut oil has for stabilizing your glucose level is that this leads directly to helping your body avoid developing diabetes. Indeed, this is good news!

In the next chapter I discuss how coconut oil can aid in keeping your teeth and gums healthy. And as good as that news sounds, the miraculous implications has for your heart health is even more exciting.

Chapter 5: Coconut Oil Pulling

When I first heard this term, I was intrigued to say the least. How do you pull coconut oil, anyway, I thought. And even if you could (and when I initially heard about this I doubted it was possible) why would anyone want to do it? So many questions flooded my mind.

I'm going to take some of the questions I had and answer them for you, one at a time. First, you're no doubt wondering what coconut oil pulling is. No, it's nothing like going to a good old-fashioned taffy pull, where you pull the candy until you get the texture you want.

I want to clear the confusion up right from the start. Many individuals learn about this practice and believe it's one of the latest fads. Nothing could be farther from the truth. And the truth is that

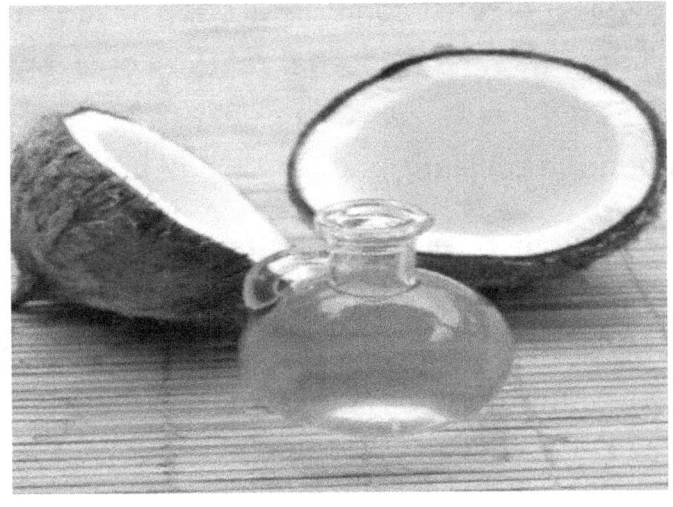

oil pulling began thousands of years ago as part of the widely revered Eastern practice of Ayurvedic medicine. It makes sense.

The traditional method uses sesame oil, but the intent is the same. People were searching for methods to keep their mouths and teeth healthy. And they couldn't just run down to the corner drug or grocery store and buy a tube of toothpaste. Even though in our society both toothpaste and tooth floss are readily available, the tradition has been handed down all these centuries, thanks to the devotees of Ayurvedic medicine.

The revival of this ancient practice couldn't come at a better time, according to some individuals. The medical community is learning more everyday about the intimate link between the health of your teeth and gums and heart disease.

At its simplest, oil pulling is the "swishing" of approximately one teaspoon of coconut oil around in your mouth. The purpose: it's simply another method of cleansing your teeth to use in conjunction with your daily hygiene ritual, to be used in addition to brushing your teeth and flossing.

Even though it's done right alongside the other two, more conventional, methods of mouth cleansing, you want to ensure that you do it properly so you can get as much of bacteria out of your mouth as possible.

Does this routine sound familiar? It's close to what you probably already do with a chemically based mouth wash. Only you're pulling this oil for a longer period of time – like for twenty minutes at a session.

You'll notice that as you "swish," the oil changes in appearance and texture. The coconut oil turns milk white the longer it stays in your mouth and mixes with your saliva. The oil, you'll notice also becomes thinner the longer you "swish."

When both of these changes take place, it's time to simply "swish" the oil out of your mouth. Be sure not to swallow this. If you do, you'll just be swallowing all the bacteria you spent twenty minutes trying to eliminate from your mouth. Now what good would that do?

The attachment of the bacteria to the oil and saliva mixture is partially why the coconut oil changes its appearance and texture. But that's not the only thing this process does. It also retards the growth of plaque in your teeth.

You can immediately see the health benefits to this discipline. It definitely reduces your risk of developing gum disease and tooth decay. But, in addition, to all of that, coconut oil pulling also helps to make your teeth whiter and stronger.

Practicing Oil Pulling

When you first begin this process, you'll notice just how long twenty minutes really is. If, in your first few attempts, you simply can't continue for the full twenty minutes, don't worry!

Few of us were able to do this in the beginning. It's definitely a habit that you gradually introduce to your system.

Start with however long you believe you can hold out at first. But do be sure to keep track of the time. The following day add another thirty seconds to a minute to this. Even if you can't do this, try to spend as much time on this ritual as you can. At the very least you're building a routine. Be patient with yourself, you'll find that you'll incrementally increase the time you "swish" almost unconsciously.

Another rule of thumb is not to "swish" this oil around your mouth vigorously, even if you know you're not going to be able to spend twenty minutes doing it. There's just no need to do it. What's more important is that you get the oil around the entire mouth. Make sure you get that oil in all the "nooks and crannies" of your teeth.

Take your time. If it helps, consider coconut oil pulling a different type of meditation. Take everything slowly, feel the texture the oil has on your mouth. Imagine the oil actually capturing the microscopic bacteria and enveloping them in that oil and saliva mixture so they have no place to go.

As previous mentioned at the end of your twenty-minute "meditation," your coconut oil and saliva mixture should be white. Spit it out and rinse your mouth with water. I can't repeat this often enough: Don't swallow this.

This, above all, is the most crucial step of the entire process. Some individuals are so adamant about not allowing any bacteria in their mouth for the moment that they actually rinse with distilled water which is void of any bacteria. Technically, that's not necessary, but the choice is totally up to you.

When your coconut-oil pulling routine is completed, then merely brush and floss your teeth as usual.

Comfort is an Issue

Hmm. Think about it. You're "stuck" swishing coconut oil around your mouth for twenty minutes at a time? Does it remind you of any other ritual you may be able do at the same try. Meditation. If you believe you can somehow incorporate the two – more power to you. I've already referred to this practice as a meditation of sorts

If you even have an inkling that you'll be incorporating this into a meditation, then you'll want to ensure that you're comfortable. If you can't get comfortable, even if you forego this as a routine meditation session, you're not very likely to do this on a regular basis.

Before you seriously begin, decide if you're approaching this as a formal meditation. Even if you bypass the meditation aspect of the ritual, you'll still be far better off finding someplace where you can get comfortable for the length of time. It'll just be easier to do.

In meditation, following your breath is a large part of the routine. It looms large as a reason why it proves to be so relaxing. In any good meditation session, start with your breath. As you sit down to pull the oil, inhale a deep breath. Do this slowly and smoothly. And remember to breathe through your nose.

You'll want to exhale at that same slow, breath, making sure once again you breathe through your nose.

When to Expect to See a Change

Many of my friends initially laughed at me when I told them what I was doing. Their first question was, "so how do you know that it's even working?" That's a good question.

Some of them assumed that I was being duped into doing something "stupid" simply because *they* had never heard of it before. Rest assured, though, that you'll see results and you'll see them rather quickly.

Within two weeks, I noticed that my teeth were whiter. At the end of a month, about four weeks time, other people (even those who thought my new-found process was stupid) noticed my whiter teeth.

Should you be plagued with gum disease, especially that which reveals itself in bleeding gums, then you'll be pleased to know that it takes about the same amount of time to help clear that up as well. After about two to three weeks of coconut oil pulling, I realized that my gums were no longer tender and didn't bleed.

Not only that, but I also realized my teeth were stronger. I consider this improvement in my dental hygiene a near miracle. I thought nothing would help strengthen my teeth again. I was prepared to get them pulled.

Oil Pulling – Not Just About Mouth Health

Would it surprise you to learn that oil pulling, for all of its amazing benefit to your teeth and gums can play an even bigger role in your overall health? It's true! Upon learning about all of these "extended benefits" of coconut oil, it finally dawned on me that that health is truly holistic. Nothing happens in our body in isolation. Consider the following healthy consequences you're setting up your body for once you begin – and maintain – the coconut-pulling oil ritual.

1. Heart Health

If you've at all kept up with the latest medical news, this may not be quite so surprising. The medical community continues to research the link between a healthy mouth of teeth and a solid and vigorous heart.

Advocates of this practice say that the theory behind this is practically self-explanatory. After all, they point out, the coconut oil contains wonderful antibacterial properties, which naturally target a wide range of bacteria, including *streptococcus.* This specific bacteria are the cause of much of the inflammation many individuals find around not only their hearts, but some arteries as well.

Because you're ridding your body of the bacteria even before it has the chance to enter your bloodstream, you're miles ahead in the health game. And you didn't even have to swallow the coconut oil itself.

2. Migraine Headaches

A greatly deliberating disorder, individuals have spent more days off work and stuck in bed because of migraines. If you're lucky enough to be able to treat them before they fully develop, that's great. But too often than not the onset of this intense, agonizing pain blind sides us.

For some individuals, it literally "blind sides" them. One of the symptoms that's characteristic of this kind of headache is a sensitivity to light. Sight is painful. Many of these individuals spend hours, if not days, secluded in a darkened room.

Vomiting is another symptom of a severe migraine headache. For some, living a normal life during the course of a migraine attack is simply impossible.

I know many individuals who began the practice of coconut oil pulling simply on the off chance that it might alleviate, even a little bit, their migraine headaches. Imagine their joy when that's exactly what happened. Not only are many individuals now living with less severe migraine pain, but they're living with fewer migraines as well.

3. Joint and Bone Pain

On the surface you may be rubbing your chin wondering why coconut pulling would even begin to show up in fewer aches and pains in not only your joints and bones, but even in your muscles.

Once you give it a little thought, the logic behind this falls into place. We're talking about oil, right? And oil, regardless of whether it goes into your body or your car, does one job very well. And that's to lubricate other substances.

Pain in your joints usually means that there's bone on bone moving inside your body, indicating that somehow your body has lost some of its natural fluids. The pain, if you've ever paid attention, also is usually accompanied by inflammation.

Most of us learned a long time ago to recognize inflammation as a bad thing. But it's really not "bad," it's merely how your body rushes to respond to pain. The fluid floods to the area of injury and this portion of your body swells – or gets inflamed. The fluid and inflammation is a protective mechanism that your body hopes will protect that area from experiencing any more pain.

That's the upside of all of this internal manoeuvring. The down side? The fluid and swelling restrict the joint's range of motion.

Arthritis is the supreme example of this process at work. This all-too-common condition does exactly this.

Even though you're not applying the coconut oil directly to the area of pain. And even though you're not even ingesting this oil, you're going to discover this wonderful side benefit. At first, you'll be tempted to call it a coincidence. Don't. Once again, everything works together in your body to give you an exciting holistic healing.

Coconut oil pulling is one of the lesser known uses of this marvelous gift of nature. Thankfully, more individuals are discovering its myriad of benefits (we've only touched the surface here!). Once you've tried it out for yourself, you'll know why.

By now, you're probably ready to get started on using this elixir of health. In fact, you may have already gone to your local health food store only to stand in front of the shelf, not knowing which type of oil would be the most appropriate for your needs. Follow me to the next chapter, where you'll learn about the varieties of oil and their uses.

Chapter 6: Types of Oil in a (Coco)Nut Shell

"I'm convinced! I'm sure coconut oil would improve my health, my hair and my skin. I even went to several stores to buy it," my friend told me not too long ago, "but . . . "

"But, what?" I asked.

"But I gave up. There are so many types of coconut oil on the grocery and health food shelves that I just gave up even before I began. I had no idea what the differences were and which would be best for my purposes."

Perhaps this is your story too. You've heard your friends rave about the near miraculous restorative health powers of 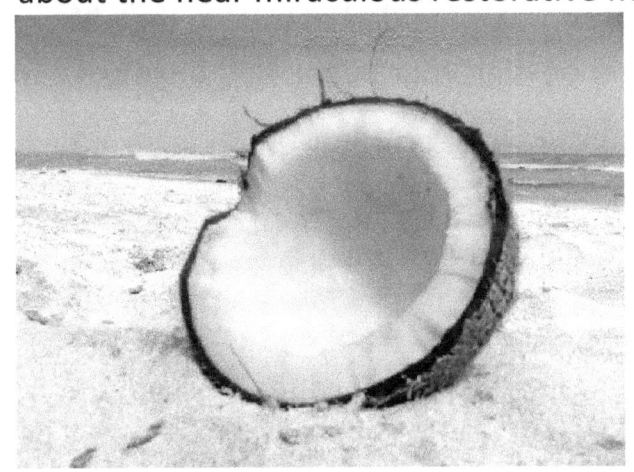 coconut oil. You've even witnessed these same individuals practically transform their health right before your very eyes.

But when you go to the store you have

what seems to be an overwhelming number of types of coconut oil to choose from. You've even tried to search the internet, only to find each site you click on is trying to sell you something. You're just not sure you can trust it.

Well, it sounded like a good idea, you mumble and continue to live your sluggish life, praying for some answer to your personal energy and health issues.

Not all Coconut Oil is Created Equal

It's true! Of course you'd expect differences in the qualities among the different brands on the market. But there are also inherent differences in the way this oil is made. Today, you're likely to find differences in the way they're processed. And yes, most definitely the specific processing procedures the oil undergoes makes a different in how they're used.

I'm here to help you navigate through the jungle of differences in this healthy oil. I promise you an impartial tour of the oils as well as their strengths in boosting your health and beauty.

Before we go through that, though, let's talk about a process that every type of coconut oil must undergo in order to get into your pantry. That's the extracting process.

It's a simple concept, really. The method of extraction is the determining variable regarding the classification of coconut oil. The better quality of extraction methods used, the higher quality of coconut oil is produced.

What exactly does "better quality of extraction" mean? It means that the more nutrients you can take with the oil when you remove it from the nut itself, the more health benefits your body receives.

Speaking broadly, boiling and cold pressing are the two main procedures which define the extraction process. Of the two, the cold-pressed method is the preferred one.

Boiling coconut oil, as you might guess, requires high temperatures which leech many of the nutrients out of the oil. The cold press procedure, though, can be done in one of two ways. It can be done manually through a process commonly referred to as bullock processing or through a machine created expressly for this procedure.

It's not surprising to learn that machine process is the more common of the two. For the most part, manufacturers use either an electrical or diesel-engine driven oil mill for this purpose

Using the simplest of classifications, you can choose from eight (8) different oils, depending on your needs.

1. Pure Coconut Oil

At one time, it was thought that pure coconut oil was the only way to use this healthy substance. While it's called "pure" it still went through some processing, however slight and natural.

Derived from the plant's dried kernels, called copra, are taken to a mill to be compressed. The mill itself is powered by either bullocks or power. The oil driven by bullocks is preferred. When you hear someone describe the substance as "pure" they generally mean that the oil possesses no additives and is unrefined and crude.

"Pure" coconut oil also implies that the oil is edible. In addition, pure coconut oil can also be used as massage oil as well as an additive to your hair. It's also makes it ideal to use cosmetic products as well as medicinal and even in the industrial world.

2. Refined Coconut Oil

While this is what it's called, depending on who you speak to, it may be referred to as "RBD coconut oil." The letters stand for refined, bleached and deodorized. Sounds like it's been really run through the mill . . . (forgive the inevitable pun).

And already you can guess that it has. Oil taken from the copra using this method guarantees that it done through mechanical and chemical refining, bleaching and deodorizing. The result is oil that's thin, colorless, without a discernible odor. But more than that, the only fats which remain are the saturated variety. One of the results of this process is that it possesses a rather short shelf live.

3. Virgin coconut oil

Oil is referred to as "virgin" when it's processed using fermentation, centrifugal separation and enzymes on the fresh milk of the coconut. Refined oil, you'll recall, uses the copra of the coconut for extraction.

The virgin variety uses fresh coconut kernels instead of copra. This can be done in two separate ways. The first is a quick-drying method which uses the least amount of heat as possible with the remaining oil being pressed out through mechanical means.

The other method is called wet milling. In this process, the fresh meat of the fruit is taken out without any drying done to it.

I know it doesn't make this oil very appetizing, let along healthy, but believe it or not, it really is.

The processing procedure used produces very little or no heat at all and the extraction process is nearly chemical free. Virgin coconut oil retains the aroma the fresh coconuts as well as their taste.

4. Organic Coconut Oil

If you encounter coconut oil that's classified as "organic," then you're holding oil that's been derived from palms raised on organic compost. Just like any other food labeled like this, it's free of man-made synthetic fertilizers and insecticides. When the oil is processed, care is taken not to use any chemicals.

All of this makes organic coconut oil quite popular with consumers. While many search the labels of food to ensure the coconut oil in the products are organic, there's also a big demand for it in other areas as well.

Organic oil of this nature is widely popular with those who want this in their cosmetic products as well. You'll find it in many organic soaps, skin creams and lotions.

5. Organic Virgin Coconut Oil

Really! And this is why when my friend started looking for coconut oil she got confused. It's really not that complicated, though, to understand what organic virgin coconut oil if you take your time to think about it some.

First and foremost, it's virgin coconut oil. You'll recall that means that it's refined using a process that produces virtually no heat. If any heat is generated during this procedure, it's very little.

Additionally, this organic virgin oil has been grown free from any man-made fertilizing materials and insecticides.

Organic virgin coconut oil is the finest quality of this variety you can possibly purchase. But before you go out to stock up on it, you need to know that it's also one of the most expensive of varieties. As great as it is, the high price may keep it out of reach of many health-loving individuals.

Let's face it, though. Even finding this variety of oil is pretty rare. You won't find it everywhere. Knowing this you may to consider purchasing it when you find it and your budget can afford it. But you may want to use it carefully as well.

6. Extra Virgin Coconut Oil

Really? You've got to be kidding. I can hear you now. No, I'm definitely not kidding. Before you reach for this variety, think twice. Believe it or not, of the eight varieties of coconut oil we're reviewing here this is one of the most highly controversial.

The name implies that it undergoes a refining process that even exceeds the standards we've talked about with the virgin type. In reality, though, there really are no benchmarks for setting the standard of excellence in oil labeled "extra virgin."

You can be certain when you purchase virgin coconut oil that it has been help up to high standards. You don't have that same assurance when you purchase the extra virgin type.

But that's not the only red flag that's waved with this label. Sad to say, those companies who not only manufacture but sell this type of oil usually are not . . . well, let's say the most reputable you can find.

7. Hydrogenated Coconut Oil

This oil is considered refined. In addition to that, the oil has also undergone a second process as well. The production of this type of oil involves the addition of extra hydrogen to the RBD oil.

So what does this mean? It means that it contains more saturated fat, the unhealthy type typically found in animal fats.

Manufacturers add the extra hydrogen in order to add to the shelf life of this oil. In a nutshell, it can sit on your grocer's shelf longer without going rancid.

If you have any doubt about whether the oil you have in your hand is hydrogenated, simply give it a good visual examination. If it's a semi-solid at room temperature, then the chances are very high that's it's hydrogenated and contains more saturated fat than the other varieties.

It's unlikely, though, that you'll discover it alongside other bottles of coconut oil. It's a product that many food producers love to use in commercially made breads, cookies, biscuits and a wide variety of other foods. This is exactly when the long shelf life of the oil is vital. It helps to keep the food product from spoiling too quickly.

8. Fractionated Coconut Oil

Even those of you who are accustomed to the other varieties of oils listed here may not be familiar with the fractionated version. It is, after all, one of the latest entrants the various types of coconut oil.

As you might guess from its name, this type of oil doesn't contain all the nutrients and molecules the other versions do. It actually contains only a "fraction" the triglycerides. It's done in such a way that it leaves this variety very heavy on the saturated fats with very few of the other types of essential fatty acids remaining.

If you were a grocer, this would be to your advantage. It means that it could give your product a much longer shelf life. But health benefits? Not as many. In fact, you probably shouldn't even use this type of coconut oil for internal.

You'll discover that fractionated coconut oil is used, more often than not, in soaps.

This saturation gives it a very, very long shelf life and greatly increased stability. It's fractionated coconut that's more often than not used for medicinal uses.

Now that you've gained a little more confidence not only in the benefits of coconut oil as well as how it's made, you're probably seriously considering using it. The following two chapters help you discover new and exciting ways to incorporate it in your daily health and beauty routine.

Chapter 7: 20 Ways Coconut Oil Can Improve Your Health

I distinctly remember the very first bottle of coconut oil I bought. (Yes, many people have told me I really need to get a life.) I had the oil in my hands. I had the potential to change my life for the better. But I wasn't quite sure how to do it. While throughout the book, I've given you examples of use, which you may have already adopted, there are so many more ways to improve, especially, your health.

This chapter provides you with twenty ways to boost your health through the use of coconut oil. Some of the methods

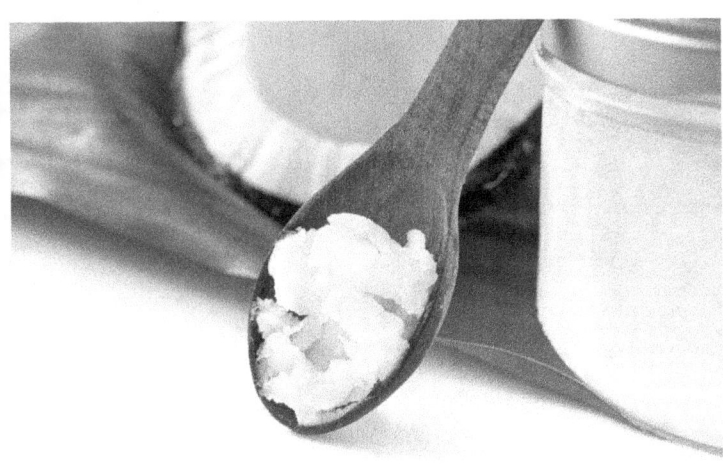

are creative. Some are obvious. All of them, however, are practical.

I've listed these in order to give you a good start on using coconut oil.

Now, you don't have to be repeating my experience – holding a bottle of the oil and not exactly sure how to use it.

Easy Ways to Make it a Habit

1. As a Cooking Oil.

With its high smoke point – the highest temperature before the oil begins to smoke and potentially burn the food – coconut oil can easily be substituted for any other oil. Whether you're using olive oil or vegetable oil, try turning to coconut oil when you're reaching for that cooking oil.

2. Take one to two tablespoons as part of breakfast or another meal or snack daily.

Put a small amount in your cottage cheese or oatmeal every morning. With its nutty flavor, this certainly won't be a chore and you won't feel as if you're downing a weight loss supplement.

3. Use it as coffee creamer

Yes, you definitely read that right. I, too, was a bit timid about this, but one of my friends encouraged me to give it a try.

(Especially after I complained I don't eat oatmeal or cottage cheese and couldn't get the oil like that.)

Needless to say I was more than a little put off by the idea, but I gave it a try. Much to my surprise, I loved it. Today, it's the only way I'll drink my coffee.

4. Nursing mothers can increase their milk supply

Nursing? Many new moms are deeply disappointed because their bodies can't produce enough milk to sustain the health of their hungry newborns. But it's been found that a breast-feeding mom can take between three and four tablespoons of coconut oil daily along with a vitamin D supplement.

This will help increase the availability of milk for your baby and you'll have peace of mind knowing that she's getting all the nutrients she needs.

5. Mix with chia seeds for all-day energy

Take a tablespoon of coconut oil and another tablespoon of chia seeds. Mix these well. Now drink it. This is a great suggestion if you know you're looking at a difficult day ahead of you. This combination is guaranteed to give you a sustained all-day energy boost.

There's just one warning here. You don't want to drink this in the evening or right before bedtime for obvious reasons.

6. Oil Pulling

We've talked about oil pulling previously as an amazing method of improving your dental hygiene and in the process your overall health. If you have any oregano add it to the coconut oil, it'll help in the healing or preventing of gum disease.

7. Use coconut oil in tea, to increase recovery time from a cold or the flu.

All it takes is a tablespoon of coconut oil into a cup of hot tea. Drink it completely and you'll start feeling the effects of a speedy recovery. Who among us can afford to take too much time off when we're sick?

8. Use coconut oil to season cast-iron skillets

If you have cast-iron skillets, you already know how important it is to season them. When you use coconut oil, you're automatically creating a layer of nutrients for your next cooking venture.

9. Use coconut oil in a homemade vapor rub recipe.

At one time or another we've all experienced the healing power of a good "vapor rub" that helps to loosen coughs. All you need to do is to rub this on your chest – or on your children's chests. Have you ever thought of including coconut oil to help hasten that healing?

This could be exactly what your body is craving to get back to good health. Below is a quick recipe for one. This differs from the commercial rubs in one crucial way, it contains no petroleum jelly.

Coconut Oil-Based "Vapor Rub"

Ingredients:

½ cup coconut oil

2 level tablespoons of beeswax pastilles

20 drops of Eucalyptus Oil

20 drops Peppermint Oil

10 drops Rosemary Oil

Directions:

1. Melt the beeswax. You can either use a double boiler if you'd like or just carefully melt it in a pan.

2. Add the essential oils and the coconut oil. If you're creating this vapor rub for a small child or infant then you want to reduce the amount of essential oils by half.

3. Stir these ingredients well.

4. Pour into a container with a lid. In fact, you might want to divide this mixture into small tins with lids. In this way you can carry one with you whenever a cough should strike.

10. Improve digestion with one single tablespoon of coconut oil before you eat.

Prior to each meal, take one tablespoon of coconut oil. This'll help ease your digestive system. It won't be long before you begin to notice a big difference in how you feel.

11. "A quick fix" to heartburn and nausea with ginger tea.

Absolutely. I've used this one many times myself. All you need to do is mix one tablespoon of coconut oil with a cup of warm ginger tea. Between the ginger and the oil, the combination will ease that heartburn and stop the nausea quickly.

12. Coconut oil can be used as a natural treatment for babies with thrush.

If you have a newborn you want to use natural products on her whenever possible. If you can avoid harsh prescription drugs or synthetic chemicals that may eventually harm your child, you're willing to go to great lengths to do.

Well, thankfully making sure your baby is receiving the most natural treatments and care is now at your fingertips.

More mothers than ever before are discovering the healing power of coconut oil for thrush. As a mom who is nursing, you have two options of treating your baby. First, you can rub the oil on your nipples so your baby's lips will connect with the oil. Alternatively, you can simply put a small amount of the oil directly onto your child's lips.

13. Coconut Oil Butter

An enjoyable way to boost your nutrients with coconut oil. Want all the nutrients and health benefits of coconut oil in a quick and easy convenient snack? Here's an effortless recipe that will have your entire family will enjoy. If you don't tell them, they'll never know how healthy this snack is.

Don't worry. With only three ingredients, this nutritious snack is easier to make than you can ever imagine.

Coconut Oil Butter

Ingredients:

1 cup of shredded coconut or coconut flakes

2-3 tablespoons of coconut oil

Optional ingredients – used according to your personal taste:

Vanilla extract

Chopped nuts

Raisins

Cocoa powder

Chia seeds

Directions:

1. In a food processor or blender, "pulse" the shredded coconut or flakes. Initially, the coconut will look like powder. Eventually it will become sticky before it turns smooth, resembling the texture of almond butter.

2. Once it thickens, add 2 to 3 tablespoons of the coconut oil and continue blending until it turns smooth again.

3. Add the optional flavorings to your tastes.

4. Continue mixing, but this time by hand.

5. Store this butter in a jar with a lid. You can store it in the refrigerator if you'd like, but it's not necessary.

6. You may want to use divide this into small jars, so it's easy to take with you regardless of where you go. Good nutrition and an energy boost will always be at your fingertips.

14. Treat urinary tract infections with coconut oil

That's right! Thanks to the nutrient-dense composition of coconut oil and its other amazing natural ingredients, it can be a natural remedy for this all-too-common infection. You can either use a bit more in your diet during the time you're experiencing this condition or you can use the oil topically.

15. Used topically to alleviate pain of hemorrhoids.

It's not an easy topic to talk about, but it is a fact of life for some of us: hemorrhoids. You could reach for over-the-counter remedies some of which are stuffed with harsh chemicals that are nearly unpronounceable.

But why do that when coconut oil can help alleviate your pain naturally? Dab some on the hemorrhoids themselves. Before you know, your pain will be greatly alleviated.

16. Add coconut oil to your smoothies

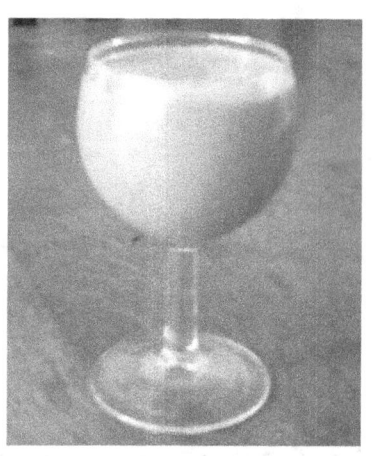

Remember that mixture of coconut oil and chia seeds we talked about for extra energy throughout the day? Why not give your morning smoothie a boost by adding just a tablespoon or two of coconut oil. You're sure to experience the sustained energy throughout your day – regardless of how long the day lasts!

But there's another advantage to this secret ingredient: you're receiving a concentration of vitamins and minerals that would be difficult to duplicate with your ordinary smoothie ingredients.

17. Apply to cold sores at the first sign of distress

You're no stranger to cold sores. They're not only unsightly, they can be painful – especially in their initial, burgeoning state. And you know what that first tingling sensation means all too well. Another cold sore.

You know by the time you find "something" to put on it, you may have already waited too long. To keep cold sores from developing, they usually demand immediate attention. Instead of running to the store, covering your mouth all the way, why not just reach into your kitchen pantry?

You guessed it, coconut oil to the rescue. When you can treat the cold sore this early naturally, then the chances are greatly improved that the sore will pop and become "weepy."

There's only one suggestion: Apply coconut oil with a cotton swap, not with your finger. If you use your finger, you're only increasing the risk of spending the virus.

18. On Your Morning Toast

That's right! Instead of using butter, or worse yet margarine, why not try buttering your toast with coconut oil. When you use the unrefined type, you'll notice a slight coconut flavor which complements the flavor of the bread perfectly. What an easy way to get that tablespoon or so of coconut oil!

19. Chocolate Coconut Fondue, Anyone?

Who doesn't enjoy fresh fruit and dark chocolate? But who dares treat ourselves to that type of splurge? Too rich. Too many calories. Not enough nutrients.

Not any more. And it's never been easier. Here's an easy way to enjoy this delicious, nutritious treat. In a double boiler, melt one tablespoon of coconut oil with two cups of chopped dark chocolate. For this to be as healthy as possible try to get chocolate that contains 70 percent cacao. If you notice that the mixture is too tight, simply add a tad more coconut oil and store some more.

Take this chocolate mixture and pour it into a fondue pot. Now enjoy it by dipping fresh fruit, like bananas and apples.

20. Movie Theater Popcorn – At Home

That's right! Who doesn't love that popcorn that's served at every movie theater in the country? More than likely it was popped in . . . of course, coconut oil.

Ever thought of recreating that smell . .. that taste . . . at home? To make this snack the healthiest possible, start with organic popcorn kernels. Pop these in coconut oil. Now melt some extra oil and drizzle it over the snack, just like it were butter (chances are you won't be using as much coconut over for the "drizzle" action as you usually do when you use butter). Add some sea salt for a perfectly healthy snack.

Making it Personal

Your imagination is probably already reeling at the various ways in addition to these you can use coconut oil to help boost your overall health and well being. This list was never intended to be a comprehensive catalogue of ways to incorporate coconut oil into your life.

The key to making coconut oil work for you is, indeed, to make it a part of your lifestyle. It can't be an action you do now and then hoping this hit and skip method will somehow work.

Regardless of what I've presented here, the only way to incorporate coconut into your life is doing what is most comfortable for you. If you're not feeling at ease with any habit, you'll never continue it. So adopt a way or two of using this elixir then stick with it. Good health will follow quickly.

If you're searching for innovate ways to incorporating this natural health-giving oil into your beauty regime, look no farther than the next chapter. I've started you off with twenty of the most popular uses of this oil.

Chapter 8: 20 Ways to Use Coconut Oil for Healthy Skin and Hair

Have you noticed? It seems as if coconut oil is in more and more commercially made beauty products than ever before from hair conditioners to anti-aging products. If you're searching for ways you can take the best of these products – the coconut oil and leave the synthetic ingredients of the products behind, look no farther.

This chapter provides you with twenty ways you can incorporate this natural oil into your daily beauty routine. In the last chapter all the ideas revolved around the use of coconut oil as a daily supplement, taken internally. This chapter shows you topical ways coconut oil can go to work providing you with healthier skin and hair.

A Tablespoon or Two Is All you Need

Keep in mind that coconut oil is such an amazingly transformative ingredient that you only need one or two tablespoons a day.

1. Use moisturizers containing coconut oil.

Many moisturizers are now including coconut oil in their formula. While you don't have to go far to discover whether your choice contains this popular oil. It's usually clearly indicated on the front of the label. Should you have any doubts though all ns this popular oil. It's usually clearly indicated on the front of the label. Should you have any doubts, though, all you need to do is check the ingredients.

By law all ingredients, must be listed. This includes those considered active or inactive by the Federal Food and Drug Administration.This cataloguing can give you a feel for how much coconut oil is in the product.

Again, by law, the manufacturers must list the ingredients starting with the one ingredient that is the most plentiful. The means the farther up on the list the coconut oil is, the more oil is in it.

2. As a makeup remover.

Think about. Removing makeup with coconut oil means you're rubbing your skin with this nutrient-dense substance, your skin is receiving all the benefits of the oil. What an easy way to soak up vitamins and minerals.

3. As a Massage Oil

And why not? As a basic oil, it serves the purpose. Once again, you'll be rubbing all the vitamins and minerals found in this substance directly onto your skin. There's no better way to make sure your skin is getting "fed" properly. Not only that but as you rub it into your skin, you know those nutrients are being absorbed directly into your body.

But don't let it stop there. Why not play with several other essential oils to create your own delightful aroma? Need a good relaxing massage? Consider including lavender or chamomile. Are you looking for a massage to lift your spirits and get you moving for the day? Why not mix your coconut oil with a bit of peppermint essential oil. Once you begin, your imagination is all that limits you.

4. Frizz Control for your Hair

A little dab will do you. At one time that was a tag line for hair cream for men. But the same could be said about coconut oil for those who have "frizzy" hair. Dab a bit of coconut oil on your hands and rub it thoroughly through your hair. Then just comb or brush it. You'll notice the change almost instantly.

Do you know what the best part of this suggestion is? You may say the best aspect is your hair absorbing all those delicious nutrients. But, for me, it's saving lots of money on the expensive hair-care products.

5. Stimulate hair growth by rubbing it into your scalp.

Why stop with curing frizzy hair? Take that "little dab" and massage it into your scalp. This can be an effective aid to coax your hair to grow faster. How could it not work? After all, you're giving your body an extra dose of nutrients to grow on.

6. Use as a hand lotion to avoid dry skin.

It's a quick fix to help keep your hands moist. If you miss the fragrance that accompanies some of the commercially bought lotions, just add your choice of essential oils to it. The advantage to doing this is that you're also adding to its soothing, moisturizing power.

7. Natural wrinkle reducer

It's almost as if coconut oil were made especially to help reduce the wrinkles around your eyes. You'll agree with me as soon as you start using it. You'll also agree undoubtedly that's it's probably one of the easiest ways to battle the initial signs of pre-mature aging.

Using a cotton ball, place the oil on the wrinkles around your eyes. Allow this to soak in overnight. When you wake up, dare to look in the mirror. Looking pretty refreshed, now aren't you?

Want to add to that look? Just add a bit of frankincense oil. After a week or so using this routine, you're sure to get plenty of compliments.

8. Heal Your Skin with Coconut Oil and Epsom Salts

There's no doubt about it, your skin takes a lot of abuse. Frigid cold in the winter, too much sun at times in the summer and an onslaught of toxins and allergens all year long. There's no way you can change that, but you can do something to help protect your skin and temper some of that damage. It's called a Coconut Oil-Epsom Salt bath. Draw your nightly bath. Add a quarter cup of Epsom salts and the same amount of coconut oil to the bath. Ease yourself into this and . . . relax. Take a deep breath.

Want to make this event extra special? Add a few drops of your favorite essential oil aroma to this.

This is a powerful combination working for you. The Epsom salts flush out the accumulation of toxins from your skin and the healing, soothing action of the coconut oil is sure to bring a sense of serenity to a stressful day.

9. Coconut Oil-Based Toothpaste

You've already been introduced to the amazing cleansing action of coconut oil pulling, but why stop there? Why not brush your teeth with a paste which includes this amazing oil?

Think of it. Not only do you receive the cleansing power of coconut oil on your teeth, but you've gained peace of mind knowing exactly what ingredients are in your toothpaste – because you placed them there.

The basic recipe is easy enough to make too! You take equal parts of coconut oil and baking soda and mix well. You can see how this is going to be pasty already. Then to make the mixture a bit more palatable to your taste buds, add several drops of peppermint essential oil into the mixture. Now stir well. You'll want to store this in a jar with lid ideally.

10. Coconut Oil based antibiotic ointment

It's no secret that coconut oil possesses definite antibacterial properties. After all, those very properties are the bases of coconut oil pulling. Including this oil in a homemade toothpaste couldn't be anything but beneficial.

So let's take it to the next level. Why not make your very own antibiotic ointment using this versatile oil?

Residents of the tropics have been using coconut oil in this fashion for thousands of years. The result? Faster healing of wounds, rashes and burns. The antibacterial and antifungal action of the oil work to keep the area of the wound or burn infection free while its lauric acid content speeds the healing.

And it really takes no time at all to mix all the ingredients together. All you need are coconut oil, frankincense, lavender and melaleuca oils.

11. Acne Clearing Ointment

It's not just the bane of teen agers, acne is a serious skin problem for millions of adults as well. The causes, as far as the medical community can detect at this point, is the overabundance of bacteria or an imbalance of the oil on the skin.

In either case, you can see how coconut oil and its diverse healing and balancing properties can be of service. When you use this oil on your acne, you're allowing its natural antibiotic traits to go to work. The oil attacks and kills the bacteria that lead to the eventual breakout.

But don't use this marvelous oil alone. If you team it up with tea tree oil and raw honey, you've just made a natural acne ointment that's hard to beat.

12. Reduces Stretch Marks

All too many women complain about stretch marks during pregnancy. The stomach grows so fast in such a short amount of time that the skin loses some if its elasticity once the baby is born. Try rubbing coconut oil on your stomach. And not just after the baby is born. You can start to rub this oil on you even before they appear. The oil works because it keeps the skin hydrated while going to work at helping the discoloration and redness and dark marks to a minimum.

13. Clean hairbrushes naturally

Why not use the cleansing and antibacterial power of coconut oil on cleaning your hairbrushes.

Merely rub it on your brushes. Don't use them for the next two hours. This ensures they're fully disinfected. After that two-hour window, then you wash them thoroughly. Don't worry though if you believe you didn't get all the oil off. After all, the coconut oil is healthy for your hair as well. Any stray oil left on the brush could only help your hair health.

14. Use as a highlight on your cheekbones.

Don't laugh! Many women are now turning to coconut oil for a natural shine to their cheeks and eye lids. It's an amazingly simple method to acquire a youthful, radiant glow without the harsh chemicals of make up. It's also costs a lot less!

15. Skin Exfoliator

Yep, making this to keep your skin looking youthful and bright is much easier than you can ever imagine. Combine coconut oil with organic coconut sugar to make a facial and body scrub with the "oomph" to remove dry skin.

Don't have any organic coconut sugar in the kitchen? Then try dry coffee grounds as a substitute. It works just as well. Try using this facial scrub even as few times as twice a week and you'll notice a big difference in your looks. Your friends will notice the difference as well.

16. Use Coconut Oil as a Sunscreen

Yes, coconut oil is an effective sunscreen and costs only a fraction of what commercial sunscreen lotions cost. With an SPF of 4, your skin is getting the protection it needs. Apply it as soon as you begin to sunbathe or start your day, and continue to re-apply it as the day goes on. That's one of the advantages of coconut oil sunscreen: it's difficult to get too much of it.

17. Relieve Painful Sunburn

You didn't put coconut oil on the last time you spent a day out in the sun. And you came home with . . . well, what did you expect: a sunburn.

Not to worry! Not only does coconut oil work as a sunscreen, but it's also an effective sunburn reliever as well. If you happen to stay in the sun too long and unintentionally find yourself burned, don't turn to commercial remedies. The oil promotes not only quick healing power, but also helps to sooth the burning sensation.

18. Natural Refreshing Coconut Oil Shaving Cream

Consider this a moment, before you toss the idea aside. You have nothing to lose by trying coconut oil as shaving cream at least once. This idea should be especially attractive to you if you suffer from razor burns or ingrown hair. Now is the time to use coconut oil as your personal shaving cream.

Warm up a small dollop of the oil in the palm of your hands (This is as easy as rubbing your hands together.) then rub this onto the area of your body you'll be shaving. Then . . . well, shave! Not only will get a smooth shave but you'll also feel totally refreshed.

19. Cellulite, Be Gone!

It's stubborn. It's unsightly. It's cellulite. But now you can battle this skin issue with a natural mixture of coconut oil. Mix one tablespoon of coconut oil with ten drops of grapefruit essential oil. Using circular motions, firmly massage this into your skin.

After you've massaged the area, dry brush it as well. This second part helps to stimulate your circulation which contributes to essential cellular detox.

20. Coconut Oil Lip Balm

Chapped lips don't just happen in the winter. They can plague you all year round. While you can rely on commercially made products, why do you want to subject your body, especially your lips, to potentially harmful synthetic ingredients?

Using coconut oil as a lip balm helps to not only nourish the lips, but also gives them some protection from the sun at the same time.

Here is all you need to do:

In a non-stick sauce pan, mix two tablespoons of coconut oil with two tablespoons of beeswax and one tablespoon of Shea butter. Warm this mixture slowly until it's melted. Be careful not to burn it. Use a small funnel and refill old, empty lip balm containers. Allow at least six hours for these to harden.

Personalize Your Use of Coconut Oil

This list of uses, just like the one in the previous chapter is simply a jumping-off point for your own creation of imaginative ways to use coconut oil topically to create healthier hair and clearer, more radiant skin.

Remember, the health of your hair and skin is absolutely an accurate reflection of your inner health.

Conclusion: The Natural Road to Health

If this book happens to be your first step into the world of natural health, congratulations! You've chosen a marvelous tool as your first venture into freeing yourself from synthetic ingredients, potentially cancer-causing agents and even

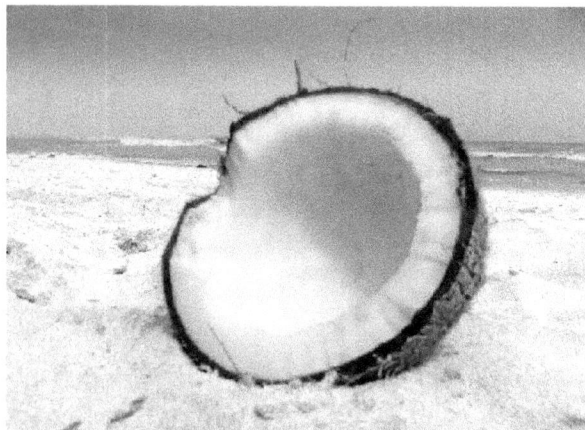

potentially damaging, harsh prescription drugs.

If you've already been using other forms of natural health products you'll discover that coconut oil is a natural addition to your already established health regime.

Either way, when you continue using coconut oil for an extended amount of time, you'll see how healthy you can truly be.

This book covers a wide range of topics. Let's get one thing straight. In no way did I write this book as a replacement for regular consultations with your personal health care provider. Anytime you change your health regime you should inform your family doctor or medical adviser immediately.

If you're taking prescription medications, he'll be able to tell you if the supplement you wish to take will interact with your current medications.

He'll also have a better idea of whether your latest choice of health supplement can really live up the claims. Does the dietary supplement work or is the publicity nothing but hype.

I also must emphasize I wrote this book not to level a diagnosis against anyone's health. If you read something in this book you believe might apply to you, again, it's up to you to step up and visit your doctor. Find out what your symptoms mean, if anything.

Once you've talked to your doctor about your use of coconut oil, then it's time to investigate why it works and decide for yourself if it will work for you.

Not all products are guaranteed to work for everyone, but the odds are this mild-tasting and health-giving oil, will help lead you to a life of robust health and vigorous, long lasting energy.

Hopefully, you'll also discover just how easy using coconut oil can be. It's the ease of use and the potential great benefits that make coconut oil such a highly popular supplement.

You only have one question you need to ask: Is it a regime that you'll find yourself following day after day, week after week?

Congratulations on your initial steps on your journey to a dazzling healthy life!